Free Yourself From Incontinence:

Your Bladder Guide

Free Yourself From Incontinence:

Your Bladder Guide

Susan L. Jackson, PT

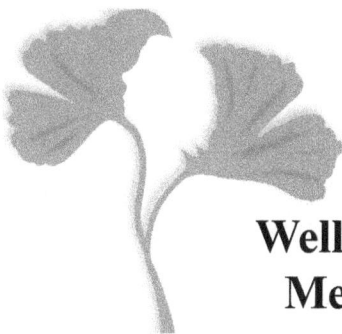

Wellness Forward
Melbourne, FL

ACKNOWLEDGEMENTS

Many supporters helped me put together *Free Yourself From Incontinence: Your Bladder Guide.* The initial idea to write the book came from working with my patients. Seeing what women could accomplish with a little knowledge and guidance, and how happy they were with the results, inspired me to want to reach more women. Thank you to all my patients for sharing your lives with me and enriching mine.

Thank you to Dr. Carolyn Fausnaugh who is the best business and bootstrapping mentor, teacher, friend, and homework assigner. I have learned much from her and look forward to learning more.

Thank you to Christine Schnitzer who was always there to bounce around ideas and lend assistance.

Thank you Linda Cobb for the feedback, support, and resources.

A special thanks to Al Curtis, former hospital administrator and friend, who was a big supporter of my work as a physical therapist and of me personally. You are fondly remembered.

Thank you to the many friends and colleagues who volunteered their time to read and comment on my rough drafts.

Thank you to the many women whose enthusiastic support of *Free Yourself From Incontinence: Your Bladder Guide* spurred me to keep writing.

CONTENTS

PREFACE

This book is to help women regain control over a problem that may be affecting their lives to cause emotional distress and diminished freedom.

The method in this book will help women take charge over the problem of incontinence so they can once again move about life freely, without embarrassment. It will also save the expense of pads and other adult protective garments. More importantly women will not have to run to the bathroom so often. My method, if followed, will have significant results. This treatment works! Women get better easily and quickly!

This book educates women about incontinence, shows them what to do, and gives them guidance to get started. Soon my patients tell me their bladder issues are improving! Great! I love helping people.

If treating this condition is such an easy task, and patients typically get great results, why do half of all Americans with incontinence never ask their doctors about it? Why would anyone choose not to get help that is readily available for such an embarrassing and freedom-limiting problem which affects 25 million women in daily life?

Many women don't realize there is a solution, and often easy solutions at that! I can't tell you how many women have expressed their surprise to me that there are treatments for incontinence beyond surgery and drugs. Many patients were also surprised at how quickly and easily their symptoms began to go away.

Many women tell themselves it's a natural part of aging. "I'm just getting old!" But is it just aging? This book challenges that belief!

For those of you who are the caregiver of a family member with incontinence, the simple exercises presented in these pages may help. The advice on controlling the urge to urinate may be something your family member can try. You may want to give your family member this book to read. Keep in mind that sometimes even well-meaning advice from a relative is not received as well as the advice from an objective professional. Especially if memory is an issue for your family member, you will need to seek the help of a professional. We are here to help!

FOREWARD

Dr. Rosemary D. Laird, geriatrician, internist, and
Medical Director of Health First Aging Institute,
Melbourne, Florida

Wouldn't you agree that urinary incontinence ranks high on the list of topics no one wants to talk about? Fortunately, Ms. Jackson isn't afraid of talking about this delicate topic. She's been inspired by the women she's helped over the years, and now fills this manual with the knowledge and strategies you can use to truly change your life. The saying that "knowledge is power" really applies to urinary incontinence. Once you understand the how and why of urinary incontinence, it becomes clear that it is possible to decrease urinary incontinence. With knowledge, you become more powerful to take steps on your own, to partner with your physicians, and ultimately make better decisions about the range of treatment options available.

In this manual, you will arrive at a deeper understanding of the anatomy of the urinary tract and the changes aging, childbirth, and illness contribute to incontinence. Notice I've listed aging, childbirth, and illness as possible co-conspirators leading to incontinence. It is not simply aging alone. While some age-related changes contribute to urinary incontinence, it is not an inevitable and untreatable effect of reaching your 65th or 85th or 105th birthday! Numerous other factors, some of which are under your control, impact urinary incontinence. For example, some incontinence is caused by what, when, and how much you choose to drink.

As you move through this manual, you will complete a thorough personal review of your dietary, urinary, related health conditions, and physical activity habits that may impact urinary incontinence.

Ms. Jackson provides sound advice with a good balance between self-help tips and working with your physician to understand the cause and factors that may be adding additional distress. The same is true of how to treat and decrease incontinence; Ms. Jackson provides a combination of self-help dietary and lifestyle modifications, paired with a recommendation to seek out information from your personal physician about the medical and/or surgical therapies that can lead most women to decreased urinary incontinence. Along the way, checklists and charting tools are provided to help guide and track your progress. This is invaluable information to bring along to your medical appointment, and will help make the most of your time with your physician.

As a geriatrician, my energies are focused on identifying physiologic changes and health conditions that negatively impact the quality of life of my patients. Urinary incontinence is a frequent culprit, robbing my patients of precious freedom to enjoy their days.

I look forward to having patients use this book. With *Free Yourself From Incontinence: Your Bladder Guide* and Ms. Jackson as their personal urinary incontinence coach, I am confident many readers will have success at decreasing the burden of incontinence.

YOU ARE NOT ALONE

Who is affected by urinary incontinence? The National Institutes of Health (NIH) reports that 26 million Americans suffer from urinary incontinence with 20 million of these being women and only 6 million men. You are not alone here. It may be that the very friends and family that you hide your problem from are hiding their problem from you.

It's estimated that Americans with incontinence spend somewhere between $50 and $1000 each year for protection from pads and on extra laundry.

If you think incontinence is just for the old, you're wrong. A review of research studies in the Annals of Internal Medicine states that urinary incontinence affect 19% of women ages 19-44, 25% of those 45-64, and 30% of those 65 and older.

Embarrassment and fear are often major concerns for sufferers of urinary incontinence. Typical worries include fear of leaking while out, concern that an odor will be noticeable or a wet spot will be visible, and not being able to return home in time. Taking pads along, making sure you wear enough protection and have enough stored in your purse are daily concerns. Decisions abut leaving home, how far to go, how long to stay, and who is with you are all affected by your desire to hide the problem. Knowing that a bathroom is conveniently located and easy to get to influences your decision of where to go, how to spend your time, and whether you go at all.

You may assume you have to accept the problem as a fact of aging, thinking that it can't be improved, or that expensive surgery or drugs are required to improve it. Maybe you're like the women who have tried kegel exercises and don't feel they've worked. You may have decided you don't want to depend on medication to manage or to consider surgical options. So you live with the problem, not knowing simple, natural answers may help.

Your bladder problems may have started after the birth of a child. Busy with the challenges of raising a family, you may have put aside your needs, assuming your incontinence will eventually go away.

You may limit your intake of fluids to avoid leaking, reasoning that if you make less urine, you will need fewer trips to the bathroom and leak less often. This rationale may sound logical, but it is not what your health professionals advise! It is absolutely the wrong thing to do because it can cause other problems such as dehydration, a life-threatening problem at worst, and a strain on the body at best. Dehydration doesn't solve bladder problems! You will still leak! And you may leak even more often or have bigger leakages because of how you're treating your bladder.

If you are older and have difficulty walking quickly enough to get to the bathroom, you may not leave home except for the necessities such as doctors' appointments and food shopping. However, as you limit activities, your physical ability to leave your home can worsen. It's the problem of "If you don't use it, you lose it." Muscles can lose strength and flexibility, and balance can worsen just because of less activity.

Losing the ability to walk longer distances than you do in your home and to stand or walk for a longer period of time results in a homebound existence. Soon follows the inability to leave your home without another person's help.

Incontinence can lead to falls at home when older women rush to get to the bathroom quickly, forgetting their walker or cane or ignoring their impaired balance. Falls at home can cause serious consequences – fractures, surgical repair of fractures, the beginning of walker or cane use, and even admission to a nursing home.

Being older and unable to leave home easily means an increased likelihood of needing help from a family member or a paid caregiver in order to continue to live independently at home.

If the incontinence is severe, it can cause an extra burden on family caregivers. When the problem becomes too severe and hygiene becomes an issue, your physician and family may consider placement in a nursing home. In fact, incontinence and dementia are the leading causes of admission to a nursing home.

NORMAL BLADDER FUNCTION

What is normal bladder function? Experts vary on how often one should urinate. ('Void' is the medical term.) Most give a range of every three to four hours. How long the stream of urine flows is important, too. Dribbling or urinating a very small amount is a sign that you are going too often. A long output of urine signals the bladder is functioning well, it has been able to collect and hold a good quantity of urine, and expels it all "in one sitting."

The color of urine is an important clue. Light yellow or nearly clear urine signals a healthier bladder. Be aware that B vitamins are excreted in the urine, coloring urine a bright yellow. It's harmless, just don't be surprised by it if you take B vitamins.

The shade of yellow is important. The darker yellow the urine is, the more concentrated the urine is inside the bladder. Concentrated urine signals that there is not enough fluid intake to care for the body's needs properly. The bladder is not able to function well without enough fluid. Substances that irritate the bladder include coffee, iced tea, hot tea, chocolate, orange juice, soda, caffeine-free carbonated soda, and milk. These irritating substances are even more irritating when there is not enough water or fluid to dilute them. When this happens, the bladder responds by voiding more frequently.

Getting up at night to go to the bathroom is common but should happen no more than once a night.

What's not normal bladder function is urinating every three hours, urinating more once at night, dribbling in the toilet rather than a strong and steady stream, dark yellow.

or brownish urine, a strong odor, or painful urination

If you have to think about your bladder function when planning your daily activities, that's not normal either.

Record your bladder function below:

Color of urine:

____ Clear

____ Light yellow

____ Bright yellow

____ Dull yellow

____ Dark yellow

____ Brownish yellow

____ Dark brown

Urine flow:

____ Strong stream

____ Weak stream

____ Dribbling

Frequency of daytime trips
to the toilet:

_____ Every 4 hours or more

_____ Every 3 to 4 hours

_____ Every 2 to 3 hours

_____ Every 1 to 2 hours

_____ Every hour

_____ Less than every hour

Record your nighttime habits:

Nighttime urination:

_____Never up at night

_____Urinate only if up for some reason other than just to go to the bathroom

_____Up only 1 time at night to urinate

_____Up 2 times at night to urinate

_____Up 3 times to urinate

_____Up 4 or more times to urinate

_____Leak only if drank something too close to bedtime

_____Leak 1 time during the night

_____Leak 2 times during the night

_____Leak 3 or more times during the night

_____Leak only in the morning when getting out of bed

_____Leak first thing in the morning on the way to the bathroom

ANATOMY: WHAT DO WE NEED TO KNOW?

It's important to understand a bit about the female anatomy in order to understand how you can help improve your incontinence. Muscles support the uterus, bladder, and rectum, and it's these muscles that make up what we call "the pelvic floor."

Think of the pelvic floor as a hammock. If the material that makes up the hammock is not in good shape, the hammock sags closer to the ground. The function of the pelvic floor is to keep the uterus, bladder, and rectum in their proper places. Without adequately strong muscles, the pelvic floor sags, allowing the vagina, uterus, bladder, or rectum to drop below their normal positions.

If an organ sags or drops down below where it should be, the medical term for that is "prolapsed." Depending on which organ has dropped down or prolapsed, there is another medical term for the condition. If it is the uterus that has fallen down into the vaginal canal, it is called a "uterine prolapse." When there is no uterus and the small intestine protrudes into the vaginal canal, it is an "enterocele." The condition of the rectum leaning into the vaginal cavity is known as a "retrocele." If it's the bladder that has dropped from where it belongs, it's called a "cystocele." Sometimes an organ can drop so low as to protrude out of the vagina. You will want to understand these terms if your physician finds you have one of them.

When these structures are out of place, the bladder may not function normally. If you have one of these conditions, you may describe a feeling of heaviness or pressure in your pelvic area, a feeling of 'falling out,' a backache, or a 'lump' in your vagina.

It's important to understand that, although we don't exercise to strengthen the bladder itself, exercising the muscles that support it can make a big difference.

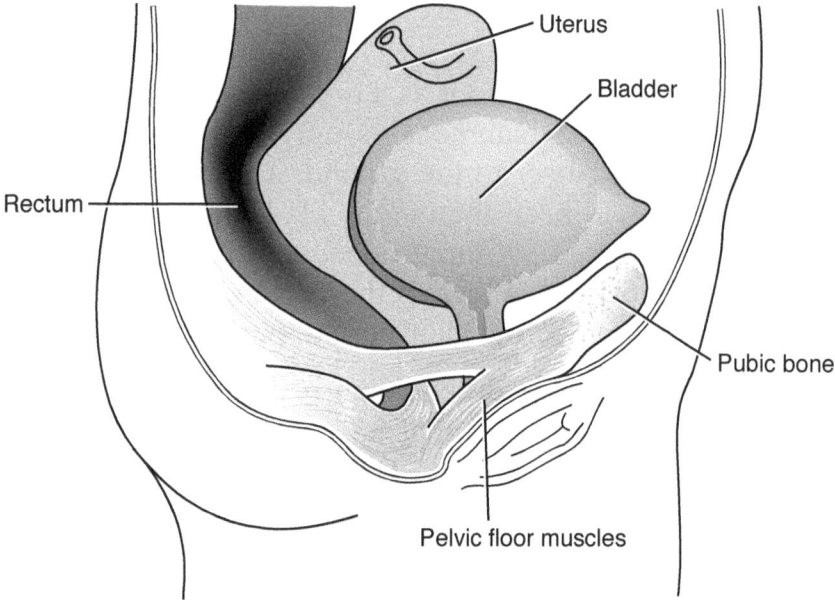

Uterus

Bladder

Rectum

Pubic bone

Pelvic floor muscles

WHAT CAUSES INCONTINENCE?

About 20 million of the 26 million or so Americans with incontinence are women. Given that fact, you can imagine that **childbirth** and menopause must play a major role in incontinence. Difficult labor, having children close together in age, having big babies, or having a lot of babies can all result in incontinence. It's the strain on the pelvic floor that does it, causing the sagging issue. Imagine the weight of baby after baby on those muscles, and all the pushing down that goes with labor. If we exercise those muscles, and tighten them up again, they can return to something close to their original condition.

With **menopause** comes many changes, including the thinning of tissues from hormonal changes. The **sphincter muscle** that stays tightly shut to keep urine from leaking may not close as well as it once did now that the tissues are thinner. That can cause a problem with urine leaking. Think of a house with a cold draft coming from underneath a non-weathersealed door, and a mother yelling, "Keep the door closed."

Bladder infections are another common problem among women. When the bladder is irritated, it seeks to get the urine out more frequently, causing increased trips to the bathroom.

A **chronic cough** is another instance of bearing down on the pelvic floor, pushing its contents downward into the vaginal canal. The frequent strain on the pelvic floor, with muscles which are already weakened, causes the bladder not to function as well. For some, the leakage may be temporary and may clear up when the cough clears up. For others, the leakage could remain, depending on how strong the pelvic floor muscles are. Keep in mind that someone with a strong pelvic floor is not likely to have leakage with a cough.

Constipation is a huge problem for many. With our diet of fast food, processed food, high sugar intake, little fiber, few fresh fruits and vegetables, limited water intake, and poor exercise habits, many experience periodic constipation. The straining that occurs with trying to relieve constipation puts a strain on pelvic floor muscles. It can cause the muscles to sag so that they don't support the bladder, uterus, and rectum adequately.

Obesity is another issue that causes excess pressure on the pelvic floor. Extra fat in the abdominal cavity can put pressure on the bladder. If you are overweight, losing just 5% to 10% of your body weight may result in fewer episodes of incontinence.

The pelvic floor muscles benefit from general exercise, so if you're already consistent with an exercise program, your pelvic floor muscles are probably in better shape than someone who does not exercise regularly. If your abdominal muscles are weak, your pelvic floor muscles are also likely to be weak. As said before, a weak pelvic floor doesn't support the bladder as well as it should, and can allow leakage of urine.

Another contributing factor is the lack of using the pelvic floor muscles naturally, as in sex. The phrase "use it or lose it" very definitely applies here. The pelvic floor muscles get exercised during the act of sex. I hope you didn't think that exercising your pelvic floor had to be boring!

Bladder irritants are those fluids and foods that cause

your bladder to leak. They include caffeine, alcohol, carbonation, citrus juices, sugar, and artificial sweeteners. Some irritants affect everyone and others affect some people more than others. If you suspect something you eat or drink causes you to be incontinent, you can take the food or drink out of your diet temporarily for a period of time to see if symptoms lessen. Try removing potential irritants for a month to give the bladder a rest, then reintroduce them into your diet one by one and note any worsening of symptoms. If a month sounds like too long, eliminate irritants for four or five days and see what happens. You can also counteract drinking an irritant you can't live without by drinking more fluid that doesn't irritate your bladder.

Caffeine, as typically found in coffee, tea, soda, and chocolate, irritates the bladder. It can concentrate urine so the bladder wants to expel that fluid as quickly as possible. Too much caffeine can cause the bladder to leak a little at a time, or to leak larger amounts. If you like your coffee, keep in mind that the more caffeine you drink in relation to other fluids, the harder on your bladder. So for you coffee lovers, if you add more water or juice to dilute the caffeine throughout the day, the better your bladder will tolerate the caffeine. Alternating a glass of water and a caffeinated beverage may help some.

What about "decaffeinated" coffee? Some say because the decaffeination process is not regulated, we don't typically know how much caffeine is left behind. Keep in mind that "decaffeinated" is not the same as "caffeine free." Some say that the decaffeination process itself leaves behind chemicals that may irritate the bladder.

Teas that are naturally caffeine free are much easier on the bladder. The best way to know if something is an irritant to the bladder is to stop drinking it for a week, then see if you notice a difference.

Carbonation is bad for the bladder. Even caffeine-free soda can be irritating. Irritation makes the bladder empty more quickly and more often. What about soda that is caffeine free and non-carbonated? Check the label. Sugar or sugar substitutes are often added, and they can be irritants too.

There's more. Citrus juices, such as orange, grapefruit, lemon, and lime also irritate the bladder when they're concentrated in the bladder. If you drink other fluids, their effect is diluted. However, if you drink only coffee and orange juice in the morning, you're more likely to have a problem in the morning.

Alcohol is a big irritation to the bladder. The more alcohol consumed, the more the irritation. Alcohol is a diuretic, just as caffeine is. A diuretic causes your kidneys to produce more urine.

At this point, most of my patients ask, "Well, what can I drink?"

"Water!"

If your reaction is "I hate water," you're not alone. Be aware that people who drink less water are more likely to have incontinence. It works opposite from what most people think.

When dealing with incontinence, many people drink fewer fluids, especially less water. What they get is an unhappy bladder with concentrated urine that can't wait to get out quickly! Also, bacteria are more likely to grow in the bladder when urine is concentrated. Bacterial growth leads to bladder infections.

I'm not suggesting you give up coffee, soda, tea, and everything else you like to drink. What I am suggesting is that you ADD some water to your day, along with the other things you drink. Only if this doesn't help should you cut out the possible offenders "cold turkey." If you are one of those who cannot bring yourself to drink water, check out the flavored waters. Read the label for sugar, artificial sweeteners, and colorings that are irritants.

Many times we may feel a craving for a soda, or another beverage, when the body is just dehydrated and needs water. Most Americans suffer from mild dehydration on a daily basis, and are not even aware of it. If you feel thirsty, you are probably already in some degree of dehydration. By drinking more water each day, your craving for other beverages will decrease.

Bladder training is another important contributor to bladder incontinence issues. If you think back to your childhood or to raising your kids, how many times did you hear, or say, "you'd better go to the bathroom just in case. We have a long car ride." How often have you gone to the bathroom "just in case?" Going when you don't really have to go trains your bladder to go more often. Or maybe you have the experience of being able to hold your urine for a long period of time when you are just too busy to go. Your bladder function is something that was trained when you were a toddler, and can be retrained now.

Do you know the possible causes of incontinence? Place a check mark by any that pertain to you:

_____ have given birth to children

_____ constipation

_____ have chronic cough

_____ have a bladder infection or frequent bladder infections

_____ are overweight

_____ have been through or are going through menopause

_____ are not physically active

_____ do not exercise

Place a check mark by any of these bladder irritants that you drink regularly:

Coffee   ___ 1 cup/day   ___ 2 cups/day
                    ___ 3 cups/day   ___ 4 cups/day
                    ___ 5 or more cups/day

Iced tea   ___ 1 glass/day   ___ 2 glasses/day
                    ___ 3 glasses/day   ___ 4 glasses/day
                    ___ 5 or more glasses/day

Hot tea   ___ 1 cup/day   ___ 2 cups/day
                    ___ 3 cups/day   ___ 4 cups/day
                    ___ 5 or more cups/day

Soda   ___ Up to 8 oz   ___ 9 to16 oz
                ___ 17 to 32 oz   ___ 33 to 64 oz
                ___ More than 64 oz

Soda without caffeine:
                ___ Up to 8 oz   ___ 9 to16 oz
                ___ 17 to 32 oz   ___ 33 to 64 oz
                ___ More than 64 oz

Soda with artificial sweetener:

___ Up to 8 oz	___ 9 to 16 oz
___ 17 to 32 oz	___ 33 to 64 oz
___ More than 64 oz	

Use artificial sweetener in your coffee or tea:

| ___ 1 packet | ___ 2 packets |
| ___ 3 or more packets | |

Citrus juice (orange or grapefruit juice):

___ 1 glass/day	___ 2 glasses/day
___ 3 glasses/day	___ 4 glasses/day
___ 5 or more glasses/day	

Milk:

___ 1 glass/day	___ 2 glasses/day
___ 3 glasses/day	___ 4 glasses/day
___ 5 or more glasses/day	

Alcohol:

| ___ 1 drink/day | ___ 2 drink/day |
| ___ 3 drink/day | |

TYPES OF INCONTINENCE

Now let's focus on the different types of incontinence. There are five basic types: stress, urge, mixed, overflow, and functional. Overactive bladder, while not incontinence, needs to be considered as well. I think it's important to understand what type you have so that you are better able to fix it!

Stress incontinence is so very common. Stress here refers to physical stress on the bladder itself, rather than emotional stress. Physical stress on the bladder causes urine to leak with activities such as laughing, coughing, sneezing, running, jumping, and/or lifting heaving objects. If the stress incontinence is really severe, it can cause the bladder to leak when you simply stand up from a sitting position. The pressure of the bladder, uterus, and rectum on the pelvic floor is less when sitting. Once standing, gravity pulls all those structures down, and the pelvic floor has to fight back to hold everything up. When you run or jump, you put even more pressure on the pelvic floor, increasing the likelihood of urine leaking.

The act of sneezing, coughing, or laughing simply puts more pressure on the pelvic floor in a downward direction. We've said that pressure downward causes weakening of the muscles and leads to leakage.

An **overactive bladder** signals the body to empty the bladder too frequently. With an overactive bladder and with urge incontinence, there is a sudden need to go. You are going about your day, when all of a sudden, you have an overwhelming need to go right now. Not later, not soon, but at this moment. The bladder muscles contract often, causing more frequent trips to the bathroom. The trigger is not physical activity as it is with stress incontinence, but the feeling of urgency.

Urge incontinence can result from an overactive bladder. Sometimes, in the medical profession, we talk about "key in the lock" syndrome. This refers to returning home from an outing and feeling the strong urge just as you put the key in the lock.

Many people leak when:

- They are trying to get to the bathroom when they first get home.
- When they get to the bathroom door.
- Standing in front of the toilet

Drugs for stress and urge incontinence are frequently advertised on television. That's because these are the most common types of incontinence. It's also common to have a combination of both stress and urge incontinence, and that is known as **mixed incontinence.**

Overflow incontinence is defined by chronically poor emptying of the bladder. It can be caused by many things, such as a neurological problem such as a stroke or MS, or a prolapsed uterus that compresses the **urethra.** Because the bladder doesn't empty fully with urination, the urine can build up and leak out. Over time, the pelvic floor muscles weaken.

You may also have a problem initiating urination. There are techniques we can teach you in person to help you deal with overflow incontinence.

Functional incontinence indicates that you have trouble getting to the toilet because of a problem with mobility, such as difficulty walking or walking slowly with a walker or cane. You may also have trouble unbuttoning, unzipping, or otherwise managing your clothes. Your balance may limit how easily and quickly you can move onto the toilet.

Problems such as these can often be improved with the help of physical or occupational therapy. Physical therapists offer specific help with balance, walking, standing up from a chair (or toilet), and more. Gaining overall muscle strength and endurance can improve functional limitations.

Occupational therapists specialize in fine motor control, including skills needed for managing buttons, zippers, and clothing. An evaluation with an occupational therapist may result in physical devices being recommended to help you get dressed and undressed easier. There may be other mobility or motor skill issues the occupational therapist will be able to improve.

It's possible to have functional incontinence yet normal bladder function, or functional incontinence along with one or more other types of incontinence.

Determine what type of incontinence you think you have and then use it as a general guideline.

My opinion as a physical therapist is, most likely, no matter what type of incontinence you have, your pelvic floor muscles are weak and will benefit from exercise. Stronger muscles almost always mean better function whether we're talking about your biceps for lifting your kids or grandkids, your triceps for lifting yourself up out of a chair, or your pelvic floor for better bladder control.

When you ask your doctor about bladder issues, be sure to mention what you think causes your symptoms. That will help your doctor begin to diagnose what type of incontinence you have. Your doctor may suggest that you see a health professional, such as a physical or occupational therapist, nurse, or nurse practitioner, who is specially trained in the treatment of urinary incontinence. Alternatively, the doctor may suggest you see a urologist or urogynocologist to have special tests run to help diagnose the problem. A urogynocologist is a doctor specially trained in both urology and gynocology for women only.

Now, check which symptoms of incontinence you are experiencing:

____ **Stress: you leak when you...**
    ___ Cough
    ___ Laugh
    ___ Sneeze
    ___ Jump
    ___ Exercise
    ___ Lift something heavy

____ **Urge: you leak when you....**
    ___ Are rushing to the bathroom
    ___ As soon as you think about going
    ___ Hear running water
    ___ Start to take your clothes down in front
        of the toilet
    ___ Put the key in the door to enter the
        house

____ **Mixed: you checked both stress and
    urge**

_____ Overflow:

_____ You don't feel like you empty your
      bladder fully

_____ You think you are finished urinating and
      then realize you're not

_____ Functional: you can't...

_____ Walk a normal pace and don't get to the
      bathroom in time

_____ Get your clothes out the way in time when
      you're in front of the toilet

_____ Balance and remove your clothes at the same
      time

_____ Get from your wheelchair to the toilet easily
      and quickly

WHAT CAN I DO ABOUT MY INCONTINENCE?

Here, I'm sharing information with you which I've shared with all the patients I've treated for incontinence. If you were to come to see me, we would talk about and try these things first. For some of you, it will be all you need to cure your incontinence.

What many women with incontinence have in common are weak pelvic floor muscles. The abdominal muscles and pelvic floor muscles haven't been used often enough to keep them in good shape. There aren't many daily activities that require the use of abdominal muscles, so they don't usually get worked without exercising them. The pelvic floor muscles, because they are internal, are used even less often. Whatever the cause of your incontinence or the type of incontinence, it is likely that weak pelvic floor muscles are a part of the problem.

Exercises to strengthen the pelvic floor will be covered in a later chapter. For now, just know that exercise is a big key to getting control over your bladder.

We've covered the effect of what you drink every day on bladder control. Later, we'll go over how to look at your typical fluid intake objectively and how to determine if it's causing some of your incontinence.

If you have urge incontinence, you will need to exercise and you will need to take a look at your fluid intake just, as those of you who have stress, mixed or overflow incontinence. However, with urge incontinence, you will also need to work on controlling the urge to go, using some simple techniques.

Let's start, first, with taking an objective look at what problems you are experiencing with your bladder control.

A BLADDER DIARY CAN HELP

The simplest tool for evaluating bladder issues is the bladder diary. The bladder diary is a record you fill out for 24 hours to 3 days, depending the health professional's preference. My patients complete a 24-hour bladder diary initially.

The bladder diary is a chart used to record the time, what you drank, when you urinated with a guess about how much, when you leaked with a guess about how much, and what activity you were doing when the leakage occurred. The words used in the descriptions in the bladder diary vary among health professionals. Some are more exacting than others in the estimates they ask of you, but the basic information is the same.

The bladder diary can tell medical professionals several things. It gives us a more objective measurement of the severity, tells where we are starting, and let's us know when we've made improvements. It also makes you more aware of potential causes of leakage. For example, this might show that your daily morning coffee habit is causing a problem. Or, you might find that not drinking enough fluids throughout the day is the problem. The bladder diary can also help you determine with certainty what type of incontinence you have.

The following examples of bladder diaries demonstrate how to fill out a bladder diary.

Example A of Bladder Diary

TIME OF DAY	WHAT I DRANK	HOW MUCH I URINATED (IN TOILET)	HOW MUCH I LEAKED	WHAT I WAS DOING WHEN I LEAKED	DID I HAVE A STRONG URGE?
06:55 am			Small	Sleeping	No
07:15 am		Small	Dribbled	Getting out of bed	
08:00 am	2 cups of coffee				
08:30 am			Small		
08:45 am		Small			
09:20 am		Small	Small	Walking to toilet	
10:15 am		Small			
11:45 am	Glass of soda				

continued

Time					
12:00 pm			Small	Walking	
12:30 pm		Small	Dribbled	Getting up from chair	
01:30 pm		Small			
02:35 pm			Dribbled	Walking	
05:30 pm	2 glasses of iced tea				
06:00 pm		Small	A lot	Walking to toilet	
07:10 pm		Small	Small	Walking to toilet	
08:00 pm			Dribbled	Sitting	
11:00 pm		Small	Dribbled	Walking to toilet	
03:00 am			Dribbled	Sleeping	
05:30 am		Small		Sleeping	

Example B of Bladder Diary

TIME OF DAY	WHAT I DRANK	HOW MUCH I URINATED (IN TOILET)	HOW MUCH I LEAKED	WHAT I WAS DOING WHEN I LEAKED	DID I HAVE A STRONG URGE?
08:15 am		Small	A lot	Running to toilet	YES!
09:00 am	Small orange juice and 1 cup of coffee				
09:15 am		Dribbled	Dribbled	Running to toilet	Yes
10:00 am		Small			
10:30 am		Small	Dribbled	Walking to toilet	Yes
11:10 am		Dribbled			
12:00 pm	1 cup of coffee				
12:25 pm		Small	Small	Walking to toilet	Yes

continued

Time					
01:40 pm		Small			
02:15 pm		Dribbled	Dribbled	Standing up	Yes
05:15 pm			Small	Arriving home	Yes
05:20 pm		Small			
06:00 pm	Glass of soda				
06:35 pm		Small			
07:40 pm		Small	Dribbled	Walking to toilet	Yes
09:30 pm		Small			
10:45 pm		Dribbled			
11:25 pm		Small			
01:05 am			Dribbled	Walking to toilet	Yes

I hope these examples help you complete your bladder diary. Notice that you need to complete every column. Being fairly accurate about the time will also help. Making a record of an entire 24-hour time period is important.

On the following page is a blank bladder diary for your convenience. Be sure to start first thing in the morning when you wake up and continue to fill it out until you wake up the next morning. You will need a 24-hour record of your fluid intake, number of trips to the bathroom, any leakage with an estimate of the amount, what you were doing when the leakage occurred, and if you had the urge.

The bladder diary is also an excellent documentation to share with your doctor or treating therapist. It will assist your health professional in evaluating your problem and recommending the next step. It's a very useful tool for us. It will easily convey a lot of important information.

When you evaluate your own bladder diary, there are several things to consider.

You may see in your bladder diary that what you are drinking is irritating your bladder. If you do, then I recommend changing what you drink for one week and to see how that affects your bladder. Continue to keep the diary to document what effect the change had.

You may also find that you need to change the timing of when you are drinking. For example, you may find that you are drinking too close to bedtime.

Maybe you'll find that urge is your biggest problem. If you are going to the bathroom frequently, then follow the tips given in a later chapter for controlling the urge.

You can also use your bladder diary to track your

progress. You might count the number of leaks you have in a 24-hour period and find that the number decreases after you do the exercises for a few days. If urge is the issue, you might find experience the urge less often.

Some people also record the number of pads used in a day. If pad usage is decreasing, that's a sure sign of progress.

Your Bladder Diary

TIME OF DAY	WHAT I DRANK	HOW MUCH I URINATED (IN TOILET)	HOW MUCH I LEAKED	WHAT I WAS DOING WHEN I LEAKED	DID I HAVE A STRONG URGE?

continued

Your Bladder Diary

TIME OF DAY	WHAT I DRANK	HOW MUCH I URINATED (IN TOILET)	HOW MUCH I LEAKED	WHAT I WAS DOING WHEN I LEAKED	DID I HAVE A STRONG URGE?

CONTROLLING THE URGE

Babies are not born with bladder control. It's a skill which must be practiced and learned. It takes time and effort to master. At first, frequent trips to the potty are needed until the ability to hold urine longer is learned.

Just as the bladder can be trained to empty on command, it can be trained to empty too often. We all sometimes go to the bathroom "just in case." Before leaving home, before a long car ride, and before a meeting are examples of when we want to be sure our bladders will not need to be emptied at an inconvenient time. We can inadvertently train the bladder to signal us to urinate before it is full.

An overactive bladder empties too frequently. The overactive bladder sends out a signal of fullness much more often than a normally functioning bladder does. The bladder is not full but there is a feeling of needing to rush to the bathroom.

An overactive bladder may lead to incontinence. The desire to empty the bladder may be so overwhelming that there is not enough time to walk to the bathroom before leaking. The problem may be small, with a dribble of urine, or it may be big enough to soak your clothes. It can lead to the feeling of your day being controlled by the urge to urinate.

Since urgency and frequency of urination are learned behaviors, the bladder can be retrained to wait for longer periods of time between emptying.

Considering what bladder irritants may be part of your daily diet is a good idea since bladder irritants can cause increased urgency and frequency of urination. Try eliminating bladder irritants and see if anything changes.

It sounds too easy, but this approach works for many people and is worth your willingness to try it.

The first thing you want to do when you feel the urge is to STOP! No more rushing to the bathroom.

When the urge comes, relax and sit down if you can. Concentrate on your breathing, taking deep breaths, think about your breathing or something else calming. Think about anything but the urge you are feeling. When the urge has passed, then stand up and walk to the bathroom. Do not run.

This is the first step. Learn to relax and control the urge rather than panic, rush, and give in to it. Do this each time you have the urge, then go ahead and get to the bathroom. You will soon be on your way to better control.

The next step, once you're comfortable with knowing you can relax and wait a bit, is to consider how long you can suppress the urge.

If you're going very often, you may only be able to work on waiting 2 minutes or 5 minutes at first. Once you're successful with that, increase the time you wait. Increase the time in increments with which you are comfortable. That might be 5-minute increments or you might feel you can jump to 15-minute increments. You're in charge of your progress here.

Regaining control of your bladder makes a huge difference in your life. It's worth the effort! Working your way toward going every 3 hours is a good goal.

EXERCISES

Exercise helps us stay healthy, independent, and feeling good. It strengthens and tones our muscles, giving us more stability, ease of movement and stamina for our daily lives. It helps us manage stress. We can use exercise to prevent, control, and sometimes even cure health issues.

This chapter will cover exercises specific to strengthening the pelvic floor as well as general exercises that provide overall strengthening that also benefit the pelvic floor resilience.

Kegel Exercises (or Kegels)

Most women have heard of kegels. Kegels is just a shorthand way of saying kegel exercises or pelvic floor exercises. Many women do not do kegels on a regular basis. Of those who know about kegels, many do not know how to do them correctly. Performing kegels the wrong way can WORSEN your incontinence, so we must be sure to get this right!

Too many women think that performing a kegel exercise means sitting on the toilet, urinating, and then stopping the stream of urine. Wrong! Stopping the flow of urine while urinating may allow identification of the muscles used to perform a kegel, but it is not the exercise itself. Performing a kegel frequently in this way can cause you to have a problem with initiating the stream of urine. It's important not to do anything to make the problem worse, so please don't do this.

Kegels are best taught one-on-one, in person. Here I

am giving you instructions on how to do kegels properly because I know there are so many of you who need help.

To do them correctly, follow the instructions carefully. Consider asking your healthcare professional to check to see that you are performing the kegel properly. This professional could be your gynecologist or the nurse practitioner in the gynecologist's office. It could be someone who specializes in the treatment of urinary incontinence, such as a physical therapist, occupational therapist, or nurse practitioner. Please don't be embarrassed. Do it for yourself, to get the control you want over incontinence.

To perform a kegel, lift up the pelvic floor slightly. There will be no outward sign that you are doing kegels.

Start working on kegels lying on your back on your bed without distractions. Concentrate on the feeling and the internal movement the kegel may produce. The pelvic floor muscles will not have to work as hard to contract in a lying position compared to sitting or standing.

To do a kegel, think of lifting up the vagina and pelvic floor. Feel like you are about to pass gas and are trying hard not to, or like you need to urinate and are trying to hold it. When performing a kegel, you should NOT feel yourself pushing down the way you do when you have a bowel movement.

If you cannot feel a slight internal motion or any sensation when you try to do a kegel, the muscles are probably too weak for you to contract them fully at first.

If the muscle contraction is so weak you barely feel it, stick with it. Perform enough kegels consistently and you should feel the contraction getting stronger. This is a great sign that you are on the right track.

After several repetitions on one occasion, or repetitions done over several days, the muscles might wake up and start to work better so you feel some control over them. If you can't feel them after 20 repetitions or even a few days of repeated repetitions, try some of the other exercises in a later chapter.

How many kegels should you do and how often?

Ten or twenty repetitions is a good start for the first day, then add 10 or 20 more each day until you can do a total of 80 kegels in one day. Continue to do the 80 repetitions until your incontinence has improved to where you want it to be, and you have been doing the kegels every day for at least 30 days.

Some research has shown that 80 repetitions a day is the best number of reps to strengthen the muscles, whereas other research has found improvement by doing fewer repetitions. If you're serious about getting results, I'd opt for working up to doing 80 a day.

"Eighty?!" I can hear you thinking it! I know it sounds like a lot, but if you think about how long it takes to do these, you'll see you don't have to invest a lot of time. You don't have to go to the gym or even walk in your neighborhood on a rainy day to do these. The privacy of your home will do. It's quick and easy once you learn how.

There's no need to do all the repetitions in one exercise session during the day in the beginning. For example, spread it out, doing 20 each time you exercise. Then, once the muscles are stronger, it will be easier to do them all at one time.

Frequently, the question comes up about when it's alright

to spread out the exercises throughout the day and when it's best to do all the repetitions and all the exercises in one session once a day. When strengthening a muscle, the more it is worked at one time, the stronger it will get. This is true of general exercise as well as kegels. The purpose of spreading repetitions or exercises out into sessions throughout the day is that the muscles are too weak to do enough in one session.

Kegels can make you feel achy in your abdominal area because you haven't been using those muscles and now they're having to do some work. If you spread out the repetitions at first, you may avoid achiness.

Once the bladder is functioning at an acceptable level, so many repetitions won't be needed to maintain that level. The number of kegels performed in a day can be decreased.

How will you know how many repetitions to cut back to? When decreasing the repetitions, pay attention to whether the symptoms begin to creep back. If your bladder starts acting up again, you'll know you can't cut back quite so much, at least not yet.

How long should you hold each kegel?

One of the best ways to exercise the pelvic floor is to strengthen both the "fast twitch" and "slow twitch" muscle fibers. All muscles have two types of fibers. Fast twitch fibers help us to move quickly. Slow twitch fibers help us to move longer with more endurance. For example, sprinting requires more fast twitch fibers, while walking long distances requires the endurance of the slow twitch muscle fibers. It's important to exercise both types of muscle fibers.

Slow kegels are typically held for ten seconds. To know how long that is, look at a clock with a second hand, or count, "1001, 1002, 1003…1010."

It's important to hold the kegel for as long as the muscles will contract. If the muscles are very weak, the hold may only last 2 seconds or 5 seconds. Start with whatever the muscles can do, increasing the length of time you hold the contraction as strength improves.

Kegels done quickly (called "quick flicks") work the fast twitch fibers by contracting and relaxing the muscles quickly. It's still a full contraction, but you don't need to count and hold it. The muscles feel sluggish at first. This should improve with exercise. If you pay attention to how it's feeling now, you'll be able to notice your progress more easily.

There's no set formula for how many kegels to do quickly and how many to do slowly. If you find you're much better at one type than the other, you may benefit from doing more of the one that's harder to perform. A good starting place might be 15 slow contractions for every 5 quick ones.

If it sounds like too much effort to do the kegels daily, think about all the women who have cured their incontinence with just kegel exercises. You could be one of them. You can potentially be free of incontinence, pads, embarrassment, and inconvenience. Free at last!

On the following pages is a chart to use as a guide to tell you how many repetitions of kegels to do each day, how long to hold each, and how many sets to do. You can check off how the pelvic floor contractions (kegels) felt, and when you did them.

Choose a day to start, and commit to doing them daily for a full 30 days. Begin with 10 repetitions, and keep adding repetitions until you reach at least 80 repetitions. Once you have followed through with your commitment, and done the kegels DAILY for 30 DAYS, you will either see improvement in bladder incontinence, or you will know that you need more help.

My Kegel Chart

Performance:

	Day 1	Day 2	Day 3	Day 4	Day 5
Number of repetitions	10	10	10	10	10
Number of seconds to hold	5	5	5	5	5
Number of sets	1	2	2	3	3
Number of times a day	1	1	1	1	1

Strength:

Did not feel the squeeze				
Felt the squeeze				
Felt a strong squeeze				

Number of kegels I did:

My Kegel Chart

Performance:

	Day 6	Day 7	Day 8	Day 9	Day 10
Number of repetitions	15	15	15	20	20
Number of seconds to hold	5	5	8	8	8
Number of sets	3	3	3	3	3
Number of times a day	1	1	1	1	1

Strength:

Did not feel the squeeze					
Felt the squeeze					
Felt a strong squeeze					

Number of kegels I did:

My Kegel Chart

Performance:

	Day 11	Day 12	Day 13	Day 14	Day 15
Number of repetitions	20	20	30	30	30
Number of seconds to hold	8	8	8	8	10
Number of sets	3	3	2	2	2
Number of times a day	1	1	1	1	1

Strength:

Did not feel the squeeze					
Felt the squeeze					
Felt a strong squeeze					

Number of kegels I did:

My Kegel Chart

Performance:

	Day 16	Day 17	Day 18	Day 19	Day 20				
Number of repetitions	40	40	40	40	40				
Number of seconds to hold	10	10	10	10	10				
Number of sets	2	2	2	2	2				
Number of times a day	1	1	1	1	1				

Strength:

Did not feel the squeeze

Felt the squeeze

Felt a strong squeeze

Number of kegels I did:

My Kegel Chart

Performance:

	Day 21	Day 22	Day 23	Day 24	Day 25
Number of repetitions	60	60	60	60	60
Number of seconds to hold	10	10	10	10	10
Number of sets	1	1	1	1	1
Number of times a day	1	1	1	1	1

Strength:

Did not feel the squeeze					
Felt the squeeze					
Felt a strong squeeze					

Number of kegels I did:

My Kegel Chart

Performance:

	Day 26	Day 27	Day 28	Day 29	Day 30					
Number of repetitions	80	80	80	80	80					
Number of seconds to hold	10	10	10	10	10					
Number of sets	1	1	1	1	1					
Number of times a day	1	1	1	1	1					

Strength:

Did not feel the squeeze

Felt the squeeze

Felt a strong squeeze

Number of kegels I did:

Kegel Alternative Exercises

If you have trouble doing the kegel exercises, especially if you can't feel the contraction or can't tell if you're doing them correctly, it may help you to start with the following exercises.

Exercising muscles that are located close to the pelvic floor muscles can help. What results is called "overflow." The action of the stronger muscles 'overflow' to the weaker muscles and cause the weaker muscles to get some exercise, too. You're exercising the pelvic floor to some degree without consciously contracting the pelvic floor muscles. Listed here are some simple hip exercises you can try.

Bridge Exercise

Bridges can be done lying on your bed. The starting position is to lie on your back with your knees bent and feet on the bed. Lift your buttocks up off the mattress, going as high as you are comfortable. For some of you, this may be as little as an inch or two, but for others it will be 12 inches or more as pictured. Bridges work to strengthen your buttocks (also called gluteal muscles). Using the buttock muscles will cause some overflow into the pelvic floor muscles so that they get some exercise without your conscious attention.

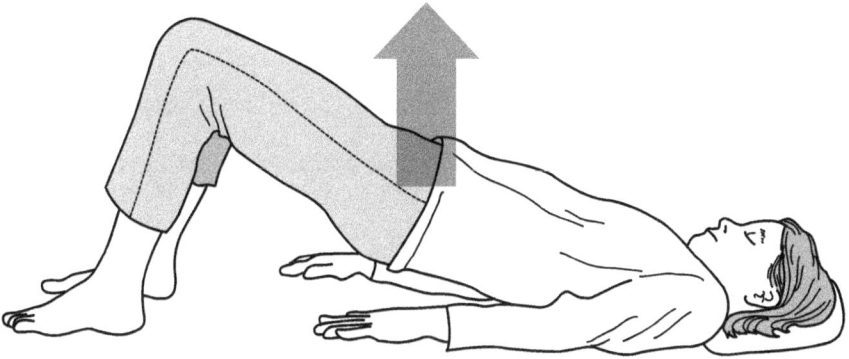

Thigh Squeezes

Inner thigh squeezes can be done sitting or lying down, depending on where you are most comfortable and are best able to exercise. If your muscles are very weak, you may find you need to lie down on your bed to do them. If you choose to sit, then sit in a chair with your feet on the floor.

Start by sitting on a chair with a 6 to 8" ball or throw pillow between your knees. Pull your pelvic floor up as you squeeze the ball between your knees. If you don't have a ball, you can use a pillow or a folded towel or blanket.

Squeeze and hold the position for a slow count of 5 (counting 1001, 1002, 1003, 1004, 1005 will give you a five-second count). Then, relax and repeat. Start with 3 sets of 10 repetitions.

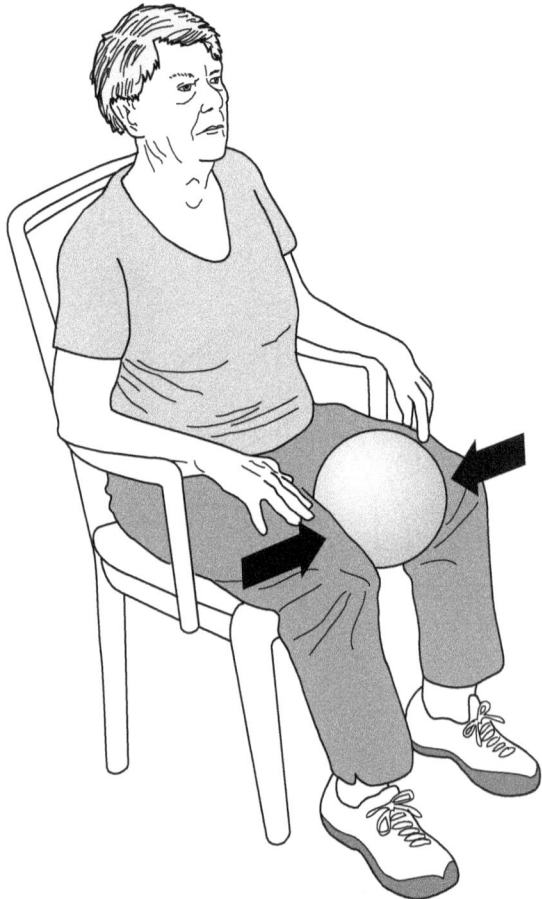

Thighs Apart

The next exercise is to bring your knees apart by working your outer thighs. You will need a stretchy band tied around legs near your knees. Bands can be purchased at most places that sell small exercise equipment such as light weights or exercise mats. They can also be found in many medical supply companies.

The color of the band indicates the amount of resistance it offers. Choose a color that corresponds to your hip strength. Ask if the resistance is light, medium, heavy, or very heavy.

Start by sitting in a chair with the stretchy band in place, first pulling your pelvic floor up and then bringing your knees apart, pushing against the resistance of the band. Do this 20 to 30 times.

If you don't have a stretchy band, push against the resistance of your hands.

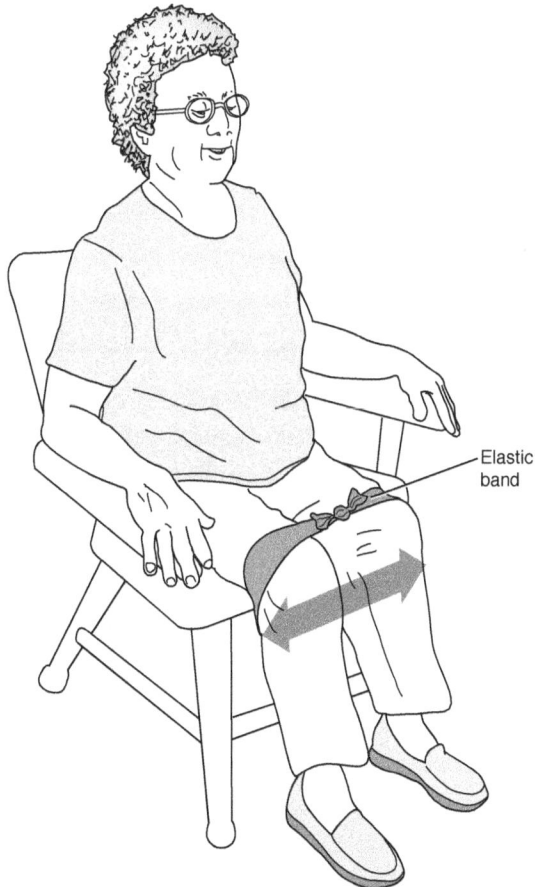

Elastic band

Abdominal Strengthening

Weak abdominal muscles can contribute to a weak pelvic floor, so strengthening these can help. The simplest abdominal exercises to do are isometrics. Sit in a chair or lie down on your back. Pull in your abdominal muscles, feeling as if you're pulling your belly button inward toward your spine, and holding it for a slow count of 5 (counting from 1001 to 1005 so that you hold long enough). Work up to 3 sets of 10 repetitions.

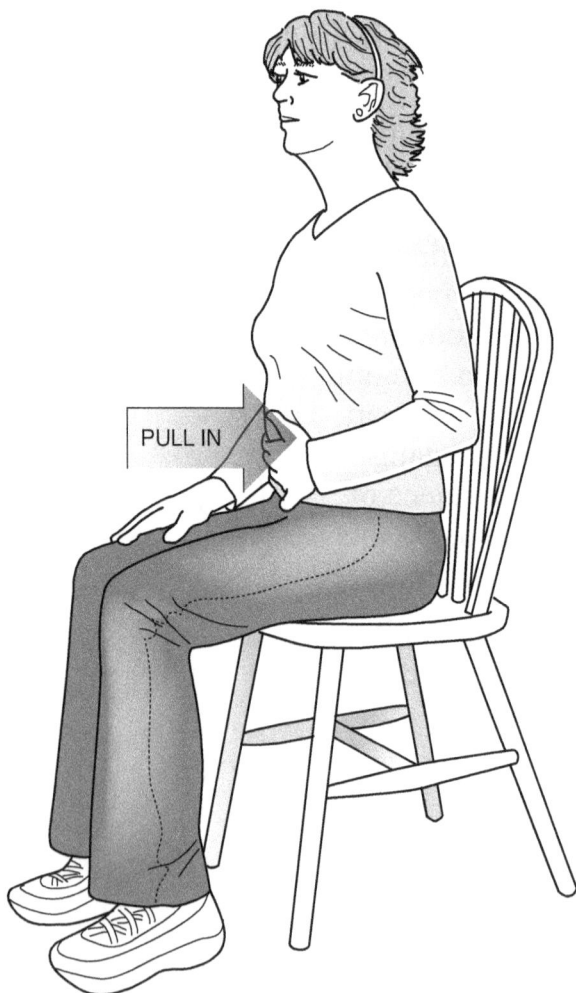

PULL IN

Walking

Walking is another exercise that can help. No special equipment is needed and no gym fees are required. Wear supportive walking shoes that fit well and offer shock absorption. If walking at night, wear clothing that is reflective and can be seen by passing cars.

Although walking doesn't specifically focus on your pelvic floor muscles, it can strengthen weak abdominals and hips which will help strengthen the pelvic floor too.

Make walking fun. Invite a friend to go along. Talking and walking is a great way to de-stress. Having a walking buddy may motivate you to get out there and be active, or you may prefer the solitude of your own thoughts.

Walk in a pretty place. Go to a park, an interesting part of town, or a pretty neighborhood.

Using a pedometer on your walk adds interest and helps track your progress. Keeping track of how many steps you take can motivate you to walk further or more often. You can also use it to count the steps you take throughout your day. You may be surprised by how many steps that is. It may help you to know that about 2,000 steps are equal to a mile.

Of course, if walking makes your symptoms worse, forget it! Try something else. There are plenty of ways to exercise. Find one that you enjoy.

Simple or Modified Yoga

Many of you may think yoga exercises are too advanced for you. Actually, beginning yoga poses are quite simple and easy.

If you are someone who has difficulty relaxing your pelvic floor muscles, this particular pose may be useful to practice and also beneficial for stress relief and overall relaxation. Here are brief instructions. More complete instructions can be found online, in a yoga book, or in a class. Take 5 minutes out of your day to lie on the floor with your arms by your sides with palms up. Start by rotating your legs in and out, and then allow them to relax gently. Allow the muscle tension in your arms to go, feeling your arms relax next to your body. Feel as if your head is pulling away in one direction and your feet and legs in the other direction. Breathe slowly and deeply as you check in with each part of your body and feel it relax.

Many poses can be modified so that they are not strenuous, but offer a gentle stretch with strengthening. That's the beauty of yoga. It offers flexibility, muscle strengthening, balance work, and relaxation all at the same time. The core strengthening provided by yoga is helpful in strengthening the pelvic floor. If you're interested in learning more about yoga, talk to the instructors in your area. Find one who is experienced in modifying poses, someone who will help you to start gently. Frequently beginning yoga classes are offered on some television stations.

More Exercise Tips

Maybe you have noticed that you feel better when you exercise. As a health professional, I know that regular exercise does make a difference. But only if you do it.

You may want to take the advice of Linda Cobb, President of The Coaching and Training Company. She advises clients to think of exercise as hygiene. It's something we must do on a regular basis because, just like brushing our teeth, it's good for us.

What I say to some of my clients is, "you don't have to like it; you just have to do it. The reward comes after the exercise, not during it."

The exercises you need to do initially to begin to get your pelvic floor into shape are not necessarily the exercises you will need to do after you've improved. This is also true in getting the rest of the body in shape. It takes more work, more time, and more repetitions to get into shape than it does to maintain it. I think of my physics lesson: a body at rest tends to stay at rest and a body in motion tends to stay in motion. It takes more energy to get the body into motion initially than it does to keep it there!

For those of you who do regular exercise but don't yet have the results that you want, re-evaluate your program. Clients often come into physical therapy and find that the exercise program they have been using is not meeting their needs. Frequently, I find that select muscles are in shape while others are not. I meet many clients who just don't know what kind of exercises they should be doing. Whether it's pelvic floor function, relief of back or neck pain, relief of shoulder or knee pain, improved balance, walking steadier without fear of falling, or anything else about your body movement, your local physical therapy clinic can advise you. Ask your physician to order physical therapy. Choose a clinic by asking your medical professional, or by talking to those who have had successful results through physical therapy.

There are a variety of activities to help you accomplish what we all really want – to feel good. Find something you enjoy, or at least something you can commit to doing consistently. Do what you need to in order get yourself moving, and to get where you want to be.

We've already talked a little about simple or modified yoga poses. Advanced or even moderate yoga provides a full body workout, offering exactly what you may be looking for – a strong core. If you are in your 60's or beyond, thinking about keeping your strength, balance, and functional mobility throughout the years to come is important. Yoga can be a great way to do that.

If you have good balance and want a bigger challenge, the fitness or stability ball also offers core strengthening. If balance is an issue for you, or if you have difficulty walking easily, don't use a ball without professional assistance. Even people who exercise regularly are sometimes hesitant to try using the big ball. If needed, a personal trainer at a gym or a physical therapist can teach you to use the ball safely.

Many gyms have stability balls available for their clients' use, and they are inexpensive to purchase for use at home. You will want to use one that fits you. You should be able to sit on the ball with your hips and knees bent to 90 degrees as if you were sitting in a chair that fits you well. Your knees should not be too high or too low. Often, stability balls come with a chart or DVD of suggested exercises. For some of you, just sitting on the ball will be a challenge. Work up to rocking on the ball side to side or forward and backward. The number of exercises you can do on a stability ball are almost limitless.

Pilates is another popular type of exercise that focuses on core strengthening. Named after the founder Joe Pilates, Pilates requires that you keep your abdomen and trunk stable while performing various exercises. Pilates are a high-level exercise for those who want to be challenged! Be sure to choose an instructor who will work with you at your fitness level.

Sports offer strengthening and conditioning while keeping the mind focused on the activity, rather than on how hard we are working! Don't be too quick to give up activities you enjoy as you raise the kids or enter the later years of life. Remember that physical therapists are specially trained to help you retain or regain physical mobility so you can continue to enjoy your daily life.

Find something you enjoy or are willing to commit to doing. Ask for any professional advice you need to get started, including talking with your physician. Getting started is the hardest part. Once you are in the routine and have some momentum going, it's easier to maintain it. You will enjoy the rewards of having a stronger, healthier body!

GETTING RID OF THOSE PADS!

Many women are reluctant to go without wearing a pad because, even though their bladder control has improved, they are not confident they can count on it. If you're feeling dependent on the pads or adult briefs, you may want to wean yourself off of the pads at some point.

Pads and adult protective garments are expensive and inconvenient to lug around. It's yet another thing to remember to buy because running out would be a problem. You have to estimate how many you'll need while out so that you have enough with you. You have to think about how to carry them discretely, and how to discard them discretely when you're out.

On the other hand, some women refuse to use pads, feeling they don't want to become dependent. This can limit how often and how long you leave home because you don't want to run the risk of leaking and being embarrassed.

I'm often asked, "How do I get away from using pads?" You may be reluctant to go without wearing a pad because, even though your bladder control has improved, you are not confident that you can count on it.

Start while you're at home. I don't expect you to risk embarrassment when you're out. If you wear a pad constantly, start by going without one for a half hour or an hour. See how it goes. You could do this for longer and longer periods of the day. Once you no longer need pads at home, try it for short periods when you are out.

If you wear a pad only when you're out, it may be scary for you to think about giving up the use of pads. You could try going out for brief trips at first, say for a drive or to a convenience store and back, to try it out and build your confidence. Take a pad with you in your purse. Keep a change of underwear and clothes in your car. Once you've proven to yourself that you can do it, pick a longer outing. Build on your success.

Whether you are lessening your dependence on the pads or getting rid of them completely, it's a freeing experience and worth the effort.

NEED MORE HELP?

If you've tried the suggestions given here, my hope is you're pleased with the results and you've regained control over your bladder rather than it controlling you. You've taken back your life.

If you've been consistent with the exercise, and can't feel the muscles contracting after a week or two of consistent exercise, you need help. Or, if you feel the muscles contracting and you've been working on it faithfully for 4 weeks without enough improvement in your symptoms, you need more help. Perhaps you need more assistance with doing the exercises correctly, more motivation, or more information. Just because you haven't gotten the results you wanted, it doesn't mean that you won't have great results with one-on-one help from a health professional.

If you feel you haven't had enough improvement in your symptoms, first ask yourself if you've given the exercises a fair chance. If you've done all you can at home, feel confident enough to ask for help, and show your doctor your bladder diary, checklists, and records.

There are more options for you. It may be as simple as getting help in doing the exercises properly, adjusting what exercises you are doing or how many repetitions. You may need more advice on controlling your urge. A specialist can offer you professional advice geared to your particular needs as well as answer your questions and offer support and guidance.

An incontinence specialist will have diagnostic and therapeutic equipment available for use in the office, such as biofeedback, electrical stimulation, or vaginal weights. Vaginal weights are light weights designed to be inserted in the vagina and held there by the pelvic floor muscles for short periods of time just as you would use a weight to strengthen your biceps. Some professionals recommend vaginal weights for some clients. They do not work for all clients.

Electrical stimulation is sometimes used when the pelvic floor muscles are too weak for you to be able to contract them yourself. The machine contracts the muscles gently, allowing the muscles to become strong enough for you to control so you can exercise them on your own.

Biofeedback is frequently used to teach kegel exercises properly. Once the machine is set up, you watch a screen to see if, when, and how strongly you are contracting your muscles. Having that feedback about what you are doing helps you to learn faster. It is also very motivating, showing you just how well your exercises are working for you. It allows you to see progress in your strength even before you see progress with your symptoms.

Know that incontinence specialists have other tests and treatments available to help. If you can't do it alone, we are here to help. There are more options available.

You are not alone!

Final Checklist

Here's your checklist to help you determine if you've done what you can on your own.

_____ Bladder irritants

    _____ Identified bladder irritants in your diet

    _____ Cut back or removed bladder
        irritants from your diet

_____ Urge control

    _____ Spent 2 weeks working on calming the
        urge

_____ Bladder diary

    _____ Completed the bladder diary for a
        full 24 hours

    _____ Was truthful and accurate in
        answering

    _____ Began the bladder diary first thing in
        the morning

    _____ Reviewed my results

____ Kegel and/or alternative exercises
    ____ Was consistent with doing the
       exercises everyday
    ____ Did the exercises for a full 30 days
    ____ Performed the exercises correctly

CONCLUSION

There is a lot you can do for your urinary incontinence. Bladder leakage is very common among women. However, it is not a normal part of aging as you might have presumed. Incontinence can occur in young women after childbirth, in middle-aged women during and after menopause, and in older women with declining physical activity. Not all women will have a problem with incontinence. Other problems such as chronic constipation, chronic cough, poor fluid intake, the wrong fluid intake, weak pelvic floor muscles, inactivity, and being overweight can contribute to incontinence at any age.

Bladder leakage is not a condition that you have to accept. It is not something that necessarily requires permanent adjustments in your life. Many women are afraid to talk to their doctor about the problem, not wanting to go on medication or have surgery. Many don't realize that there are other treatments to try before considering something invasive like surgery or medication that may cause side effects.

Exercise to strengthen the pelvic floor, general exercise for overall health, delaying the urge, or losing ten pounds are some of the approaches that can improve and even cure incontinence.

I, like other health professionals who treat urinary incontinence, have helped many women do that.

Consider the women who find that, with a little change in what they drink every day, or by spending some time to control their urge to go, they can eliminate or reduce their incontinence. Other women find that a little daily exercise makes a big difference. The practical, natural methods reviewed in *Free Yourself From Incontinence: Your Bladder Guide* have worked for many women.

If the suggestions given here don't improve your symptoms as much as you'd like, medication, appliances, and surgery are still options to be considered. Sometimes the combination of medication, diet, and exercise work best to get you started or may be necessary to continue long term. When exercise is part of the treatment, surgery is often more successful and the improvements last longer.

Consider one woman's comment that her urogyncologist had recommended surgery but she was reluctant to agree to it. After reading this book, she went through the checklist on her own. Then she spoke with her doctor about the possibility of trying a different option. She was able to get more detail from her doctor about his recommendation and her condition. He was able to tell her that her pelvic floor muscles were strong. She was able to understand, with the use of diagrams, her specific problem and his plan for correcting it surgically. After reading the book and having a more informed discussion with her doctor, she then felt good about choosing surgery.

As women, we don't want to limit our lives. We have too much to contribute to our families, our work, our world, and ourselves.

The answers are in your hands, and now you have the opportunity to take control. Take charge. Change your situation. You have the tools here. To leak or not to leak. It's all up to you.

About the Author

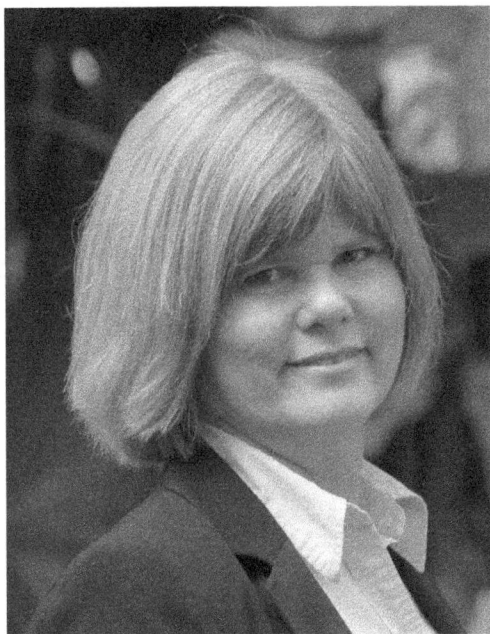

Susan L. Jackson offers more than 20 years of expertise as a Physical Therapist and Aging Expert specializing in middle age and older adults. She has a passion for empowering older adults to maintain their independence and regain lost function, as well as educating and assisting those in middle age with prevention. Ms. Jackson treats a variety of age related conditions, issues, and challenges, including urinary incontinence. Her clinical experience includes a variety of settings such as private practice, outpatient facilities, rehabilitation hospitals, and long-term care communities. She is a graduate of the University of Florida, a member of the American Physical Therapy Association's Section on Women's Health, and a member of the National Association for Continence. Ms. Jackson is available for lectures and workshops on wellness and aging topics. Contact her through her website www.bladderguide.com.

www.ingramcontent.com/pod-product-compliance
Lightning Source LLC
Chambersburg PA
CBHW030028290326
41934CB00005B/532